Somatic Therapy

Integrative Techniques for Sexual

Health, Grief Recovery, and Pain Relief

Beth James

Dedication

To all those on a journey of healing, may you find peace, strength, and connection through the wisdom of your body.

Epigraph

*"The body holds our deepest truths; it is through its wisdom
that we find our path to healing."*
— Beth James

Table of Contents

Preface

Somatic Therapy: Integrative Techniques for Sexual Health, Grief Recovery, and Pain Relief is born out of my deep passion for helping others reconnect with their bodies and heal from within. This book distills years of experience into actionable steps that anyone can take to address their physical and emotional challenges. My hope is that these practices will empower you to find balance, resilience, and well-being in your everyday life.

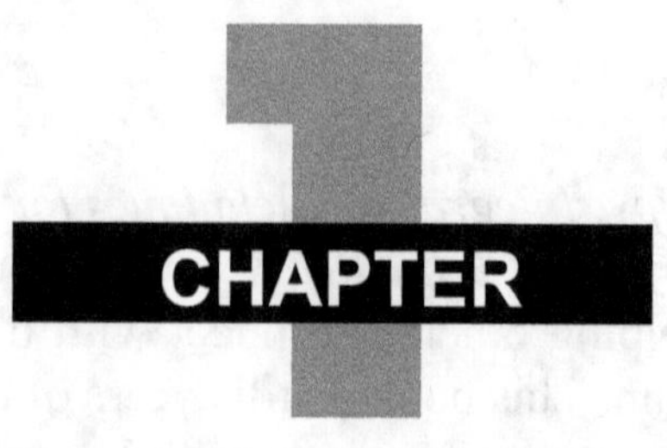

Introduction to Somatic Therapy Understanding the Mind-Body Connection

The mind-body connection forms the basis of somatic therapy. This idea shows how our mental and physical states interact. Our thoughts, emotions, and psychological states can affect our physical health. At the same time, our physical state can impact our mental well-being.

Two-Way Link Between Mind and Body

The mind and body have an impact on each other in both directions. This is based on the idea that our emotions can affect our physical state, while our physical condition can change how we feel. For example, when we feel stressed or anxious, our body might react with signs like a faster heartbeat, tight muscles, or stomach problems. Conversely, long-lasting pain or sickness can make us feel down or worried.

This link isn't just for show; it's rooted in how our bodies work. Our autonomic nervous system, which runs things like our heartbeat and digestion without thinking about it, is affected by how we feel. When we're scared or worried, the sympathetic part of this system kicks in with the "fight or flight" reaction. This leads to physical signs like a racing heart or quick shallow breaths. But when we're calm and safe, the parasympathetic part takes over with the "rest and digest" response. This puts our body and mind in a peaceful state.

Emotions Showing Up as Physical Feelings

Feelings often show up in our bodies, which is crucial to how somatic therapy works. Take sadness - you might feel a heaviness in your chest. Or anger - your jaw or fists might tighten up. These body reactions aren't random; they're tied to what's going on in our minds and hearts. Think about that "knot in your stomach" when you're worried or those "butterflies" when you're excited.

What is Somatic Therapy?

Definition and Origins

Somatic therapy, also called body-centered therapy, influences both the mind and body to tackle psychological, emotional, and physical problems. The word "somatic" comes from the Greek word "soma," which means "body." Unlike traditional psychotherapy, which often focuses on thinking and feeling aspects of mental health, somatic therapy stresses the body's role to heal.

The roots of somatic therapy go back to the early 1900s. It draws from many areas like psychoanalysis, bodywork, and Eastern practices such as yoga and meditation. Some key people shaped how somatic therapy grew. Wilhelm Reich, a psychoanalyst, looked at how holding back emotions ties to physical tension. Alexander Lowen developed bioenergetic analysis, which mixes physical exercises with talk therapy. As time passed, somatic therapy began to use ideas from brain science, trauma research, and mindfulness methods.

Core Principles of Somatic Therapy

Somatic therapy stands on a few main ideas that set it apart from other ways of helping people:

1. **Body Awareness:** Somatic therapy stresses knowing your body sensations and physical states is important. This knowledge plays a crucial role in spotting and working through emotions, trauma, and stress that hide in the body. Therapists often use deep breathing, step-by-step muscle relaxation, and body scanning to help people connect with what their body feels.

2. **Integration of Physical and Emotional Experiences:** Somatic therapy acknowledges the connection between emotional and physical experiences. Emotions don't just exist in our minds; we also feel them in our bodies. Take anxiety, for instance. It might show up as tight shoulders or a constricted chest. By combining body sensations with emotional processing, somatic therapy helps people let go of pent-up trauma and experience a more complete form of healing.

3. **Embodiment:** Embodiment means experiencing life in your body. Somatic therapy helps people reconnect with how their body feels and understand what it's trying to tell them. This can make you more

aware of yourself and better at handling emotions when things get hard. To embody yourself, you might try moving, paying attention to your senses, or picturing things in your mind.

Somatic Therapy vs. Traditional Talk Therapy

Somatic therapy and traditional talk therapy differ in what they focus on. Like cognitive-behavioral therapy (CBT) or psychodynamic therapy, talk therapy deals with the mind—thoughts, feelings, and actions. It involves talking about past events, looking at thought patterns, and working through emotional problems by talking.

Somatic therapy puts the body at the heart of the healing process. This approach believes that the body holds on to trauma and emotional pain, which can show up as physical symptoms or ongoing tension. By working with the body, somatic therapy aims to free these pent-up emotions and trauma, helping people heal from within.

Traditional talk therapy often focuses on changing how people think about and interpret their experiences—a process called cognitive restructuring. On the other hand, somatic therapy zeroes in on what's happening in the body and how it feels to help people feel safe and grounded in the here and now. This method works well for those who've gone through trauma, as it sidesteps the mental defenses that can get in the way of processing emotions.

Traditional therapy can sometimes lead people to over-analyze their problems. They might understand the issues in their head but find it hard to feel or work through their emotions. Somatic therapy takes a different approach. It encourages people to feel and let go of emotions through their bodies. This can result in a more thorough, all-encompassing healing that cares for the mind and body.

Somatic therapy is a strong, body-focused treatment method highlighting how the mind and body work together. It gives people a different way to heal by paying attention to body feelings, combining physical and emotional experiences, and encouraging people to be more in touch with their bodies.

The Role of Somatic Therapy in Holistic Healing

Addressing Physical, Emotional, and Spiritual Health

Somatic therapy influences holistic health by considering how physical, emotional, and spiritual aspects of well-being connect. While traditional therapies often focus on the mind, somatic therapy recognizes that the body stores memories of trauma, stress, and emotional experiences. To heal, this approach works with the body to release these stored experiences. This process helps to improve health in many ways.

Physical Health: Somatic therapy impacts physical health by helping people tune into their body's feelings and patterns. This better understanding lets folks spot areas where they hold tension, hurt, or feel uncomfortable. These spots link to emotional problems they haven't worked through yet. The therapy uses methods like checking in with your body, breathing exercises and moving to help loosen up tight muscles and calm down. Somatic therapy can boost overall physical health and energy by easing these body symptoms.

Emotional Health: Emotions aren't just mental experiences; people also feel them in their bodies. Somatic therapy helps people connect with these physical emotions, allowing them to work through and let go of feelings they might have pushed down or not recognized. This can lead to clearer emotions, better bouncing back from tough times, and more balance. By tackling how emotions show up in the body, somatic therapy can help folks have a more complete and true-to-themselves emotional experience.

Spiritual Health: Somatic therapy also recognizes how spiritual health matters in complete healing. It promotes a strong link with oneself, creating a feeling of inner calm, direction, and harmony. Methods like grounding, centering, and visualization help people tap into their inner knowledge and gut feelings, leading to spiritual growth and healing. This spiritual side of somatic therapy helps those looking to find deeper meaning and connections in their lives.

Somatic Techniques to Support Overall Healing and Balance

Somatic therapy uses many methods to support healing and balance in several ways:

1. **Breathwork:** Your breath can have a powerful influence on somatic therapy. Therapists use different breathing methods to help clients become more aware of how their body feels, let go of tension, and balance their nervous system. For instance, breathing from your diaphragm can soothe your mind and body, while more energetic breathwork can help you release bottled-up emotions.

2. **Body Scanning:** This method involves guiding clients to check their body from head to toe to find

areas that feel tense or uncomfortable. This practice helps to boost body awareness and often serves as a starting point to explore physical and emotional issues more.

3. **Grounding Exercises:** Grounding techniques help clients connect to their body and the present moment. These exercises include feeling their feet on the ground, focusing on their breath, or using images to link with the earth's energy. Grounding is key in making clients feel safe and stable in their bodies.

4. **Mindful Movement:** Somatic therapy often uses movement practices, like yoga, dance, or simple stretches, to help clients let go of stored tension and reconnect with their body's natural rhythms. Mindful movement encourages people to explore how their body wants to move in a gentle, accepting way. This promotes both physical and emotional release.

5. **Touch and Bodywork:** Some somatic therapy forms involve therapists using touch to help clients notice their physical feelings and emotions. This can include gentle contact or more organized bodywork based on what makes the client comfortable and what they want to achieve.

6. **Visualization and Imagery:** Therapists use visualization methods to help clients picture themselves, letting go of stress, healing hurts, or finding balance in their body. These mental exercises can change both physical and emotional states.

The Importance of a Holistic Approach to Health and Well-Being

A holistic approach to health looks at the whole person—body, mind, and spirit—instead of just treating symptoms. This approach plays a key role in somatic therapy because it sees that true healing needs to address all parts of a person's life. By combining physical, emotional, and spiritual practices, somatic therapy provides a full path to wellness.

Holistic healing recognizes that our physical problems often link to our emotional and spiritual states. For instance, long-term back pain might not just be a physical issue but could also connect to emotional stress or past trauma. Somatic therapy aims to uncover these links, allowing deeper and longer-lasting healing.

A complete approach gives people the power to play an active part in their healing journey. Clients can make smarter choices about their health and well-being by figuring out how to tune in to their bodies and grasp the signals they get. This self-knowledge and self-care result in a more balanced and rewarding life.

Somatic therapy is vital in whole-person healing, tackling the complex links between physical, emotional, and spiritual health. Through a mix of methods designed to support overall balance, somatic therapy helps people gain a more profound sense of well-being, giving them the power to live more and be true to themselves.

Enhancing Sexual Health through Somatic Techniques Common Sexual Health Issues

Sexual health plays a crucial role in overall wellness, but many common problems can affect it for both men and women. As a doctor and body-focused coach, you must understand the physical and mental factors involved in these issues.

Main Problems: Trouble Getting Hard, Low Sex Drive, and Worry About Performance

Erectile Dysfunction (ED): ED means a man can't get or keep an erection good enough for sex. Many things can cause this problem, like heart and blood vessel issues, diabetes, nerve problems, and mental stuff such as stress or worry. Looking at the body as a whole, ED isn't just about physical problems. It can also link to how a person feels old, hurts they haven't dealt with, or long-term stress, which all affect the part of the nervous system that works without us thinking about it.

Low Libido: Low libido, or less interest in sex, can stem from hormone problems, long-term illnesses, drugs, or mental issues like feeling down, worried, or having relationship troubles. In body-focused therapy, experts often look into hidden emotional blocks, stress, or old hurts that might affect someone's sex drive and energy. Methods that help people understand their bodies better and manage their feelings can work well.

Performance Anxiety: Performance anxiety is a widespread problem for men. It happens when fear of not being good enough in bed causes worry, leading to poor sexual performance. This worry can come from society's expectations, personal doubts, or bad sexual experiences in the past. Somatic therapy provides ways to stop this cycle. It helps build a stronger link between mind and body, keeps people focused on the present, and lowers the body's "fight-or-flight" response during sex.

Gender Differences in Sexual Health Issues

Sexual health problems can look different in men and women. This often happens because of differences in body function, hormones, and cultural background:

- **Men:** Guys tend to face problems like trouble getting or keeping an erection and feeling nervous about their performance in bed. These issues often tie into what society expects from men and how "manly" they should be. When men feel stressed or worried, it can make these problems worse. Body-focused therapy can help men get back in touch with how their body feels without any judgment. This can lower the effect of things that stress them out.

- **Women:** Women might deal with low sex drive, trouble reaching climax, or discomfort during sex. These problems can link to hormone shifts, like those in menopause, or mental factors such as body image concerns, past sexual trauma, or relationship issues. Body-focused therapy can help women by tackling both the emotional and physical sides of their experiences. This approach aims to ease tension and help women reconnect with their sexual selves.

Psychological and Emotional Factors Affecting Sexual Health

Mental and emotional elements have a significant impact on sexual health. Problems like stress, anxiety, depression, past trauma, and relationship troubles can all lead to sexual problems. These issues often create a loop where emotional distress causes physical symptoms, which then make the emotional distress worse.

Stress and Anxiety: Long-term stress turns on the sympathetic nervous system, which causes cortisol levels to rise. This has a negative impact on sexual desire and performance. Worrying about how well you'll do in bed can make it hard to relax and be present during sex. This leads to problems with getting aroused and feeling satisfied. Body-focused methods like staying mindful, breathing exercises, and becoming more aware of your body can help control the nervous system. These approaches lessen how much stress and anxiety affect sexual health.

Depression: Depression often causes people to lose interest in things they used to enjoy, including sex. Feeling tired and unmotivated, plus possible side effects from antidepressant drugs, can reduce sexual desire and performance even more. Somatic therapy can help people reconnect with their bodies, which can break the cycle of feeling disconnected and numb, which often comes with depression.

Past Trauma: Sexual trauma or abuse can leave lasting emotional and physical scars, leading to many sexual health problems like pain, avoiding intimacy, and trouble trusting a partner. Somatic therapy offers a safe environment to process these traumatic memories through the body, allowing people to let go of stored trauma and rebuild a positive connection with their sexuality.

Relational Dynamics: The quality of a relationship has a big influence on sexual health. Problems like poor communication, unsettled arguments, or feeling distant can lead to sexual issues. Somatic therapy helps couples to look into and boost their physical and emotional bond, often resulting in better intimacy and more satisfying sex.

Somatic Exercises for Improved Sexual Function

Enhancing Body Awareness and Sensation

As someone who teaches somatic methods, I know that getting more in touch with your body plays a big part in making sex better. This means learning to notice and pay attention to how your body feels. You can do this through some easy but powerful exercises:

1. **Body Scanning:** Start by lying down. Shut your eyes and breathe a few times. Move your focus from your toes up to your head, paying attention to different parts of your body. Take note of any spots that feel tight, relaxed, or have any other feeling without judging them. This exercise helps you get more in

tune with your body and how it reacts, which plays a key role in improving sexual function.

2. **Pelvic Floor Awareness:** Your pelvic floor has a big impact on your sex life. Find a comfy spot to sit or lie down. Focus on the muscles in your pelvic area. Try to squeeze and release these muscles. Notice how it feels. This practice makes you more aware and can make your pelvic floor stronger. This might boost your pleasure and performance in bed.

3. **Sensory Exploration:** Try exploring your senses by touching different parts of your body softly. You can do this alone or with a partner. Pay attention to how it feels and how your body reacts. This exercise helps you connect more with your body and can make you more sensitive to touch and pleasure.

Breathing Exercises to Relax and Lower Anxiety

Breathwork has a substantial impact on somatic therapy for people who feel anxious about sex. The right way to breathe can help your body and mind unwind, making it easier for you to be present in the moment.

1. **Diaphragmatic Breathing:** People also call this belly breathing. This exercise involves breathing into your diaphragm instead of taking shallow breaths into your chest. To do this, put one hand on your stomach and the other on your chest. Take a deep breath through your nose, letting your belly rise while your chest stays still. Then, breathe out through your mouth. This way of breathing turns on the parasympathetic nervous system, which helps to lower anxiety and make you feel more relaxed.

<u>**Diaphragmatic Breathing**</u>

2. **4-7-8 Breathing Technique:** This method can help to calm your nerves and lessen stage fright. Here's how it works: Breathe in through your nose while counting to 4, hold your breath for a count of 7, then breathe out through your mouth for a count of 8. Do this four times in a row. The 4-7-8 approach helps to balance your nervous system and can make you feel more relaxed and focused.

<u>**4-7-8 Breathing Technique**</u>

3. **Paired Breathing:** When you do this with a partner, paired breathing can make you feel closer and more connected. Sit so you face each other and match your breathing. One of you breathes in while the other breathes out, making a smooth back-and-forth pattern. This can help you feel in tune with each other and in the moment, which is great for intimacy.

Mindfulness Techniques to Improve Intimacy and Communication

Mindfulness is crucial in somatic practices and strongly impacts intimacy and communication between partners. To practice mindfulness means to be aware and involved in the present without judging or letting your mind wander.

1. **Mindful Touch:** Explore each other's bodies with slow, deliberate touches. Pay attention to the feelings and emotions that come up as you touch. Talk to your partner about what feels good. This exercise helps

couples slow down and value each moment, strengthening physical and emotional closeness.

2. **Loving-Kindness Meditation:** This meditation technique helps to create feelings of love and compassion, which can strengthen emotional closeness. Start by sitting in a comfortable position and concentrating on your breathing. say phrases such as "May I be happy, may I be healthy, may I be at peace." Then, extend these wishes to your significant other, picturing them and hoping for their happiness and peace. This practice can boost empathy and bonding in your relationship.

3. **Eye Gazing:** Eye gazing means partners sit face-to-face and keep eye contact for a long time. This task can be challenging but helps build trust and make emotional bonds stronger. It pushes non-verbal talk and can create a strong feeling of being connected. People find this method basic, but it has a deep impact.

These body-focused exercises aim to build a stronger bond with your physical self, lower stress, and boost closeness and talking in relationships. By making these methods part of your daily life, you can create a more satisfying and linked sexual encounter.

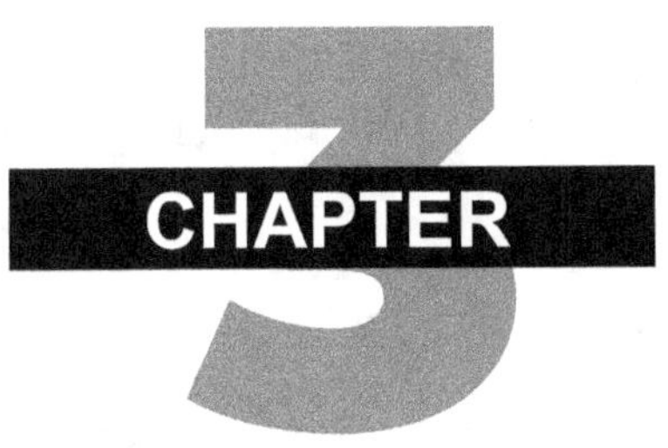

CHAPTER 3

Grief Recovery and Somatic Therapy Understanding the Grieving Process

Grief changes a person's life. It's personal and complicated. Somatic therapists need to know how grief works to help people deal with loss. This chapter looks at grief stages, how grief shows up in the body, and how loss affects mental health.

Stages of Grief According to the Kubler-Ross Model

Elisabeth Kubler-Ross came up with the Kubler-Ross model in 1969. It describes five grief stages that many people go through but are not always in order. These stages include:

1. **Denial:** People first react to loss by finding it hard to accept what's happened. Denial serves as a way for them to protect themselves, letting them come to terms with the shock.

2. **Anger:** As denial starts to fade, people might feel frustrated and helpless. They could direct this anger

at themselves, others, or even the person who died. It's key to remember that feeling angry is normal and helps with healing.

3. **Bargaining:** During this phase, people often try to strike deals or make trades to regain control or undo the loss. They might use "what if" and "if " phrases, showing how much they want to change what happened.

4. **Depression:** When the full impact of the loss sinks in, people may feel very sad and hopeless. This stage involves pulling away from others, having less energy, and feeling like nothing will ever be okay again. It's a time when someone faces how big the loss is.

5. **Acceptance:** The last stage sees people coming to grips with their loss. Acceptance doesn't mean the pain is gone, but rather that the person is figuring out how to keep going and adjust to life without their loved one.

People don't always go through these stages in a set order. They might bounce between stages or deal with several at once. Knowing about these stages helps you figure out where someone is in their grieving process and how to best help them.

How Grief Affects Your Body

Grief isn't just about feelings. It can also have an impact on your body. Some common ways it shows up are:

1. **Fatigue:** Grief can wear you out. Dealing with loss impacts your emotions, which can drain your energy.

This often leads to ongoing tiredness and a lack of drive to do things.

2. **Sleep Disturbances:** Grief often messes with sleep. You might find it hard to fall asleep, stay asleep, or get restful sleep. On the flip side, some people sleep too much to escape the hurt they're feeling.

3. **Appetite Changes:** Grief can shake up your eating habits. You might lose all interest in food, or you might overeat to comfort yourself. If you don't monitor these changes, they can affect your overall health.

4. **Somatic Complaints:** Grief often causes physical symptoms in the body. People might get headaches, stomachaches, tense muscles, or chest pain. These body aches show how emotional pain can affect us.

5. **Weakened Immune System:** Grief puts much stress on the body, making the immune system less effective. This means people who are grieving might get sick more. To stay healthy, eating well, getting enough sleep, and finding ways to handle stress during this tough time is crucial.

Emotional Impact of Loss on Mental Health

Loss has a deep effect on our emotions, and this has an impact on mental health in several ways:

1. **Depression:** The Kubler-Ross model points out that depression often shows up when people grieve. It can be as mild as feeling a bit down or as severe as clinical depression. People might feel empty inside,

lose hope, or stop caring about things they used to enjoy.

2. **Anxiety:** Losing someone or something important can make people feel anxious. They might worry about what's next, feel like everything's too much to handle, or even have panic attacks.

3. **Guilt and Regret:** Many people who grieve feel guilty or regretful. They often ask themselves if they could have done things. This self-blame can slow down their healing and make it hard to move forward.

4. **Isolation:** Grief impacts social behavior, often causing people to pull away from others. They might think no one can grasp their suffering, or they don't want to weigh others down with their feelings. This retreat can make their sense of being alone and hopeless even worse.

5. **Cognitive Impairment:** Grief also affects how the brain works. It can make it hard to focus, remember things, or make choices. This "fuzzy" state is a normal part of dealing with loss, but it can upset those going through it.

Understanding how grief affects emotions is critical to giving full-fledged help in bouncing back from loss. Body-focused therapy can be crucial to assist people in working through these feelings by tackling both the physical and emotional sides of grief.

Somatic Techniques to Process Grief and Loss

Grief has a physical impact on the body, often causing tension, pain, or feelings of detachment. The body-focused approach of somatic therapy offers practices to help people work through grief and loss. These methods aim to reconnect individuals with their bodies and release pent-up emotions. Some in-depth, educational, and engaging techniques support this process.

Body-Centered Practices: Exercises to Ground and Breathe

Grounding Exercises: Grounding is a key practice in somatic therapy to help people feel more present and linked to their bodies. When you're grieving, you often feel detached or cut off from reality. Grounding exercises aim to counter this by tying you to the here and now.

- **The 5-4-3-2-1 Exercise:** This exercise gets you to use your senses to focus on what's happening now. Start by looking for five things you can see, four things you can touch, three things you can hear, two things you can smell, and one thing you can taste. This straightforward but effective method helps you pay attention to your body and what's around you, making you feel more grounded and relaxed.

- **Feet on the Ground:** Stand or sit in a comfortable position and place your feet on the ground. Picture roots growing from your feet deep into the earth. Notice the connection with the ground and how it supports you. This practice helps lower anxiety and gives you a feeling of safety, which is key when you're grieving.

Breathing Exercises: The breath connects the mind and body, and mindful breathing greatly impacts how we feel.

Technique 1: Diaphragmatic Breathing: People also call this belly breathing. This method involves breathing into your diaphragm. Put one hand on your chest and the other on your belly. Take a deep breath through your nose, letting your belly rise while your chest stays still. Breathe out through your mouth. This way of breathing helps calm your nerves, reduce stress, and make you feel more at peace.

Technique 2: Box Breathing: This breathing method helps keep your nerves in check and can calm you down when grief hits hard. Breathe in for four counts, hold it for four, breathe out for four, then wait for another four counts before starting again. Keep this up a few times, paying attention to how your breath flows. This approach brings order and peace when your emotions are all over the place.

Breathing Exercises

Embodied Meditation and Visualization Techniques

Embodied meditation and visualization have a strong impact on somatic therapy. They help to merge the mind and body when someone grieves.

Body Scan Meditation: This meditation influences scanning the body from head to toe, bringing awareness to each body part. Begin at the top of your head and move down, noticing any tense, painful, or uncomfortable areas. Breathe into these spots, picturing the breath as a healing power that lets go of tension and brings about relaxation. This practice helps you spot where grief might appear in your body and encourages release and relaxation.

Heart-Centered Meditation: Find a comfy spot and put one or both hands on your heart. Turn your attention to your heart area. As you breathe in, picture yourself pulling in warmth, love, and kindness. When you breathe out, let go of any hurt, sadness, or stress. This way of meditating helps you be kinder to yourself and deal with the emotional pain that comes with loss.

Visualization Techniques:

Safe Place Visualization: Picture a spot where you feel safe and calm. This could be somewhere real or made up. Use all your senses to make this place come alive in your head. See yourself in this spot, soaking up the safety and comfort it gives you. This method gives you a mental hideout when grief gets too much, letting you escape for a bit and feel some peace.

Grief Release Visualization: This exercise asks you to picture your grief as something you can touch inside your body—maybe a big rock or a dark cloud.

Then, imagine you're taking this thing out of your body and letting it go into a river or the ground. As you do this, you picture your burden getting lighter and feel relieved. This can help you work through your feelings, as it shows the process of moving on in a way you can see and feel.

<u>**Visualization Techniques**</u>

Movement Therapies: Dance and Yoga to Release Emotions

Moving your body allows you to express and let go of emotions. Somatic therapy often uses movement therapies such as dance and yoga to help people work through grief.

Dance Therapy:

> **Freeform Dance:** Play music that matches how you feel and let your body move as it wants. Don't think about your appearance—focus on what you feel. Use your body to show the emotions inside you, like sadness, anger, or even happiness. This free movement helps you let go of bottled-up feelings and can make you feel free.

> **Guided Dance Ritual:** This method has a clear structure. You start by choosing a goal before you dance. Your goal could be to honor your sadness or to link up with your inner power. Pick music that matches your goal, and let this purpose guide how you move. This dance ritual can help change your grief into a solid way to heal and learn about yourself.

Yoga for Grief:

Technique 1: Heart-Opening Poses: Cobra (Bhujangasana), Bridge (Setu Bandhasana), and Camel (Ustrasana) are poses that open the heart. These postures help you let go of emotions stored in your chest. They encourage deep breathing and open up your heart chakra. This can lead to emotional release and healing.

Restorative Yoga: Restorative yoga uses props to support the body in easy, relaxing poses that need little effort. Poses like Child's Pose (Balasana) and Reclined Bound Angle Pose (Supta Baddha Konasana) calm you down and help your nervous system relax. These poses give your body a safe place to unwind and work through emotions at its own pace.

Moving Meditation: This blends easy yoga sequences with mindful breathing, enabling you to process your grief with awareness and physical involvement. Concentrating on motion and respiration helps remove mental and emotional obstacles, fostering a feeling of ease and letting go.

Using these body-focused methods in your grief healing journey can give you strong ways to handle the tricky feelings and body reactions that come with loss. These practices offer a kind physical approach to getting better, letting you work through grief in a complete and unified way.

Creating a Balanced Mind-Body Approach to Healing

Combining Somatic Therapies with Traditional Talk Therapy

To take a holistic approach to grief recovery, you should combine somatic therapies with traditional talk therapy. Talk therapy gives you a chance to process emotions and thoughts through dialogue, while somatic therapy involves the body releasing stored tensions and trauma. This two-pronged approach allows for a more thorough healing experience. When you address both the thinking and physical parts of grief, you can achieve a deeper and more complete recovery.

Take a client exploring why they feel grief in talk therapy. They spot thought patterns that add to their hurt. Then, they can try things like breathing exercises, grounding methods, or body checks to let go of how grief shows up in their body. This might be tight muscles, feeling tired, or ongoing pain. Using both types of therapy helps mind and body, giving a fuller way to heal.

Adding Spiritual Practices and Rituals to Help Healing

Spiritual practices and rituals can help when recovering from grief. When facing a loss, they can give a sense of purpose, connection, and continuity. These practices are often very personal and can be quite different based on what someone believes and their cultural background.

- **Mindful Meditation:** Adding mindfulness or meditation to daily habits can help people create a feeling of being present and calm. This allows them to connect with their inner selves and discover peace amid the chaos of grief.

- **Rituals of Remembrance:** Taking part in rituals like lighting a candle for the person who died, making a memory book, or hosting a small ceremony can offer a planned way to honor and remember loved ones. These rituals help to process emotions and can play a vital role in the journey to healing.

- **Nature Connection:** Spending time in nature can give your spirit a boost. This could mean taking a walk, working in the garden, or just sitting outside. Nature's life cycles - birth, death, and rebirth - often match our feelings. This can offer comfort and a new view when times are tough.

A Well-Rounded Strategy to Help People Heal from Loss

A strategy that considers the whole person to help people heal from loss recognizes how the mind, body, and spirit are all connected. This approach ensures that every part of a person is taken care of and nurtured as they work to get better.

- **Physical care** includes working out, eating right, and getting enough sleep. How we feel plays a big role in our emotions, and our feelings affect our physical health, too.

- **Emotional Support:** It's critical to have people to lean on and ways to express and work through feelings. This could mean attending therapy often, joining support groups, or talking with close friends and family.

- ● **Mental Health:** Writing in a journal, reading books, or making art can help keep our minds clear and focused. These activities give us a way to process our grief.

- ● **Spiritual Health:** Taking part in activities that strike a chord spiritually, be it through religious rituals, quiet reflection, or getting involved in the community, can give you a sense of meaning and help you feel connected.

By combining body-focused therapies with counseling, adding spiritual elements, and taking a full-person view, people have a better chance to heal from grief in a well-rounded way. This mixed approach doesn't just deal with the current signs of grief but also helps build long-term strength and health.

Managing Chronic Pain with Somatic Therapy
The Mind-Body Pain Connection

Chronic pain is complex and involves many aspects. Both physical and mental factors shape it. As a skilled somatic coach, you must help clients grasp how the mind and body link in pain experiences. This chapter will examine how stress and emotions affect pain perception, the brain and body processes that connect mind and body pain, and the studies showing that somatic therapy works well to manage pain.

How Stress and Emotions Affect Pain Perception

Stress and emotions greatly impact how we feel and experience pain. When we're stressed out, or our emotions are all over the place, our bodies react by turning on the sympathetic nervous system. People often call this the "fight or flight" response. This causes our bodies to release stress hormones like cortisol and adrenaline, which can make us more sensitive to pain.

For instance, stress can make your muscles tense up in your neck, back, and shoulders. This tension can make existing pain worse or even cause new aches. Pain can feel stronger and tougher to handle when you're anxious, scared, or down. This happens because negative feelings and stress can lower how much pain you can take. As a result, things that might not hurt when you're calm can become painful when stressed out.

Also, chronic stress can put the nervous system in a state of hyperarousal, where the body gets stuck in a heightened state of alertness. This state can make the body more reactive to pain signals, creating a cycle where pain causes more stress, which then increases pain.

How the Mind and Body Connect to Create Pain

The connection between mind and body pain is based on complex brain and body processes. The brain and nerves play a crucial role in how we process and feel pain. Pain signals travel from the hurt or uncomfortable area through the nerves to the brain, where the brain reads them and we feel pain.

- **Central Sensitization:** Central sensitization plays a crucial role in ongoing pain. This happens when the nervous system becomes extra sensitive, making pain signals stronger and sometimes causing pain even when there's no outside reason. We often see central sensitization in conditions like fibromyalgia and chronic fatigue syndrome, where people keep feeling pain without any clear injury to blame.

- **Neuroplasticity:** The brain can change its structure, which we call neuroplasticity. This has an impact on chronic pain. When someone feels pain for a long time, the nerve paths that carry pain signals can become more set. This makes the pain last longer. That's why pain can stick around even after the first cause improves.

- **Psychosomatic Pain:** Another key idea is psychosomatic pain. This happens when feelings or mind troubles show up as body aches. For instance, sadness that won't go away, bad memories, or worry can lead to long-lasting pain in different body parts. This pain is real but comes more from how someone feels than from a physical hurt.

Understanding these mechanisms shows why treating long-term pain requires more than just physical symptoms—it requires a complete approach that includes the mind and feelings.

Studies Supporting Somatic Therapy to Manage Pain

Somatic therapy has gained attention as an effective way to manage long-term pain by addressing both the physical and emotional parts of pain. Research in this area has shown that somatic practices can reduce pain intensity and enhance the overall life quality for people with chronic pain.

- **Mindfulness-Based Stress Reduction (MBSR):** Research shows that MBSR influences chronic pain reduction and improvement in pain-related disability. MBSR includes somatic practices like mindful movement and body awareness. This practice helps people to develop a non-judgmental awareness of their pain, which lowers the emotional distress linked to it.

- **Body Awareness Therapy:** Studies on body awareness therapy, a type of somatic therapy, suggest that it can enhance pain management. It does this by helping individuals to become more in tune with their body's signals and responses. This heightened awareness can result in more effective self-regulation and pain reduction.

- **Breathwork and Pain Perception:** Research on breathing methods, like deep belly breathing, shows that managing your breath can lessen how much pain you feel and help your body's automatic functions work better. This helps people whose pain gets worse when they're stressed or anxious.

- **Somatic Experiencing (SE):** Dr. Peter Levine created SE to treat trauma stored in the body. Studies on SE prove it works to reduce long-lasting pain when that pain is tied to past trauma or emotional issues that haven't been dealt with.

Treating long-term pain through somatic therapy requires grasping the complex link between mind and body, tackling the emotional and brain-related factors that play a role in pain, and using proven somatic methods. By mixing these approaches, people can achieve a more balanced, complete recovery from persistent pain, leading to better health and quality of life.

Somatic Approaches to Relieve Pain

Body Awareness and Mindfulness Practices to Lessen Pain

Body awareness and mindfulness serve as key methods in somatic therapy to help people handle pain. These techniques encourage individuals to focus on their body's feelings and emotional conditions. By practicing these methods, people can relax, feel less stressed, and develop a sense of comfort in their bodies. This process often leads to a noticeable decrease in how much pain they feel.

1. **Body Scan Meditation:** This method requires you to check your body bit by bit, starting at your head and ending at your toes. As you do this, you notice where you feel tight, sore, or hurt, but you don't judge these feelings. When you pay attention to these spots, you can learn to loosen up and feel less pain. This approach also helps you see how feelings like stress or worry might be making your body hurt.

Body Scan Meditation

2. **Mindful Breathing:** Concentrating on your breath helps control your nervous system and brings you a sense of calm. Methods like diaphragmatic breathing (deep belly breathing) or 4-7-8 breathing can turn on your parasympathetic nervous system, which makes you relax and feel less pain. This practice also keeps you in the present moment, which can stop your mind from worsening pain through worry or fear.

Breathing Exercises

3. **Progressive Muscle Relaxation (PMR):** PMR involves tightening and loosening different muscle groups, beginning with the feet and working your way up. This method boosts your awareness of your body and helps ease muscle tension that can add to pain. By relaxing each set of muscles, your body becomes more relaxed, which can lessen chronic pain.

Progressive Muscle Relaxation

Somatic Movement Therapies: Feldenkrais and Alexander Technique

Somatic movement therapies such as the Feldenkrais Method and the Alexander Technique have a significant impact on chronic pain management. These approaches focus on retraining the body's movement patterns and aim to enhance posture and alignment.

1. **Feldenkrais Method:** Moshe Feldenkrais created this approach. It uses soft, mindful movements to help people explore and boost their movement. The main goal is to make people more aware of how they move and teach them new, better ways to do it. The Feldenkrais Method can help lessen pain and improve overall physical function by reducing extra tension and stress.

2. **Alexander Technique:** The Alexander Technique aims to teach people how to move and hold their bodies better. It helps people learn new ways to stand, sit, and move, which can ease pain and discomfort. This method is suitable for neck, back, and shoulder pain. It shows people how to use their bodies in a balanced way, which leads to better posture and less stress on their muscles and joints. By doing this, it can help reduce long-term pain.

Exercises to Relax and Ease Muscular Tension

Exercises that relax and ease muscular tension play a crucial role in managing chronic pain through somatic therapy. These exercises help to loosen tight muscles, boost blood flow, and create a feeling of calm and wellness.

1. **Gentle Stretching:** Easy stretch exercises that focus on areas where tension builds up, like the neck, shoulders, and lower back, can loosen tight muscles and boost flexibility. Stretching as a part of your daily habit can stop tension from piling up and making pain worse.

2. **Yoga:** Yoga blends careful movement, breath control, and stretching to help you relax and feel less pain. Some poses work well to ease muscle tension and help you unwind. These include Child's Pose (Balasana), Cat-Cow (Marjaryasana-Bitilasana), and Legs-Up-the-Wall (Viparita Karani).

3. **Somatic Movement Exploration:** Try free movement or light dancing to see how your body wants to move. This natural movement helps your body let go of built-up stress and can help people who deal with long-term pain. The main thing is to

move without judging yourself, letting your body lead the way.

People can get significant pain relief from long-lasting aches by making somatic approaches a regular habit. This leads to better overall health and more control over how they feel. These techniques do more than ease the pain. They also give people the tools to connect more with their bodies, which helps healing and toughness in the long run.

Integrating Mindfulness into Pain Management

Benefits of Mindfulness Meditation for Pain Relief

Research has shown that mindfulness meditation has an impact on chronic pain management. This practice teaches people to concentrate on the now and observe sensations without judging them. As a result, it reduces the emotional and mental reactions to pain, leading to decreased pain perception. Mindfulness encourages people to accept pain, which enough, can make the pain seem less intense and overwhelming. With regular practice, mindfulness can retrain the brain to respond to pain with less reactivity and more calmness, which improves overall quality of life.

Guided Exercises in Mindful Breathing and Body Scans

Mindful Breathing: Start by sitting in a comfortable position and pay attention to your breath. Feel the air as it comes in and out of your nose, watch your chest go up and down, and notice your belly expand and shrink. When your thoughts drift away, bring your focus back to your breathing. This exercise helps calm your nerves and can make pain feel less intense.

Body Scan Meditation: Lay down or find a comfortable seat and shut your eyes. Focus on your toes, then shift your attention up your body—feet, legs, torso, arms, and head. Pay attention to any spots that feel tense, painful, or uncomfortable, and notice these feelings without trying to change them. This exercise helps you spot and release physical tension linked to pain.

Starting a Regular Mindfulness Routine to Manage Ongoing Pain

Making mindfulness a part of your daily life can significantly impact how you handle pain over time. Start small with 5–10-minute sessions of mindfulness meditation or body scans each day. As you get used to it, you can make these sessions longer. The key is to stick with it—regular mindfulness practice can change how your brain deals with pain. This can lead to less intense pain and less emotional stress from it. You can also bring mindfulness into everyday tasks, like walking or eating. This helps boost your overall mindfulness and makes it easier to manage pain.

When you make mindfulness a regular habit, you can build toughness against long-term pain. This gives you a feeling of control and boosts your overall health. This well-rounded approach doesn't just help you handle pain. It also sharpens your mind, balances your emotions, and relaxes your body. All of this adds up to a healthier, more rewarding life.

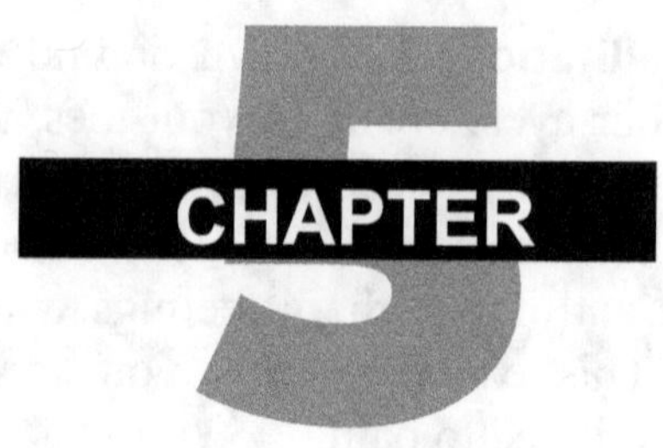

Practical Somatic Exercises and Techniques
Grounding and Centering Exercises

Grounding and centering play a key role in somatic therapy. These practices help people connect with their bodies and focus on the present. They work well to manage stress, anxiety, and strong emotions. They also create a solid base for emotional and physical health.

Techniques to Help People Feel Grounded and Centered

1. **Barefoot Grounding:** Walking barefoot on natural surfaces like grass, sand, or soil is one of the easiest and most powerful ways to ground yourself. People call this practice "earthing," and it helps you connect with the earth's energy, making you feel more stable and relaxed. As you walk, pay attention to what your feet feel—the ground's texture, how warm or cool it is, and how each step feels. This careful attention strengthens your link to the earth and can help reduce feelings of worry or being out of touch.

Barefoot Grounding

2. **Rooting Visualization:** Plant your feet on the ground, keeping them shoulder-width apart. Shut your eyes and picture roots sprouting from the bottom of your feet, reaching deep into the earth. See these roots securing you, giving you support and sustenance. As you inhale, imagine pulling up energy from the earth through your roots, and as you exhale, feel any stress or tension flowing down into the ground. This exercise helps create a strong sense of being grounded and linked to the physical world around you.

Rooting Visualization

3. **Five Senses Technique:** This grounding exercise impacts bringing your attention to your surroundings by using your five senses. Start by noticing five things you can see, four things you can touch, three things you can hear, two things you can smell, and one thing you can taste. This method helps to focus your mind on the here and now, easing anxiety and making you feel more balanced.

Five Senses Technique

Visualizations and Mental Pictures to Boost Stability

1. **Mountain Visualization:** Find a cozy spot and shut your eyes. Picture yourself as a mountain—tough, steady, and rock-solid. See your body as the mountain's base rooted and firm, with your head stretching like the peak. Sense the mountain's power and steadiness inside you. This mental image can boost your inner strength and bounce-back ability, giving you a stable mind and emotions.

<u>Mountain Visualization</u>

2. **Tree Visualization:** Like the rooting exercise, this visualization asks you to picture yourself as a tree. Plant your feet on the ground while standing or sitting. See roots growing from your feet, grounding you to the earth. Think of your body as the tree's trunk, sturdy and straight, with your arms as branches stretching out and up. Picture these branches moving in the breeze, bending but not breaking. This mental image helps you feel balanced, adaptable, and linked to your surroundings.

<u>Tree Visualization</u>

3. **Light Visualization:** Find a cozy spot to sit or lie down and shut your eyes. Picture a warm, glowing light that spreads out in the middle of your body. When you breathe in, see this light grow, filling you with warmth and calm. When you breathe out, imagine the light pushing away any bad feelings,

tension, or stress from your body. This mental picture helps create a sense of inner peace and emotional balance, grounding you in calm and steadiness.

Ways to Find Calm and Feel Better Inside

1. **Breath Awareness:** Paying attention to your breath is one of the best ways to balance your emotions. Start by sitting in a comfortable position and noticing your breath. Watch the natural rhythm of your breathing without changing it. When you breathe in, picture yourself taking in calm and peace. When you breathe out, imagine letting go of stress and tension. Practicing this often can help you manage your emotions, feel less anxious, and find inner calm.

Breath Awareness

2. **Progressive Muscle Relaxation:** This method involves tightening and loosening different muscle groups in your body, beginning with your toes and working your way up to your head. As you tighten each muscle group, breathe in, and as you let go of the tension, breathe out. This approach helps to ease physical tension and can help to manage stress and worry. The step-by-step relaxation of muscles brings a deep feeling of calm and emotional balance.

Progressive Muscle Relaxation

3. **Meditative Walking:** Meditative walking combines the perks of mindfulness and physical activity. Pick a quiet spot where you can stroll. Pay attention to each step, how your feet feel as they touch the ground and your breathing pattern. When thoughts pop up, notice them and shift your focus back to walking. This exercise helps you stay grounded, keeps your emotions in check, and creates a feeling of inner quiet and tranquility.

<u>**Walking Meditation**</u>

4. **Body Anchoring:** This method helps you focus on where your body touches the ground or a surface. Sit or lie down and pay attention to how your body feels against the chair, floor, or bed. Take note of the pressure, warmth, and support you feel. This practice makes you feel more grounded and supported when anxious or overwhelmed.

<u>**Body Anchoring**</u>

5. **Weighted Blanket Grounding:** A weighted blanket can make you feel like someone's hugging you, which can calm you down. The pressure from the blanket helps turn on your body's relaxation system, making you feel more grounded and at ease. This method works well for people who get anxious or find it hard to stay in the moment. It has a strong impact on helping them relax and feel more present.

Pictures in Your Mind for Staying Steady

1. **Anchor Visualization:** Picture yourself as a ship dropping a big heavy anchor into the ocean. See the anchor going down through the water, reaching the bottom of the sea where it digs in. As the anchor settles, you start to feel steady and peaceful. This mental image can help when things are rough, giving you a picture of being safe and stable.

Anchor Visualization

2. **Golden Light Visualization:** Picture a golden light entering your body from the top of your head. As this light moves down, see it spreading warmth and relaxation to every muscle and cell. Feel the light connecting you to the earth as it reaches your feet. This mental image helps you relax and builds your emotional strength and inner calm.

Golden Light Visualization

Ways to Find Calm and Feel Better Inside

1. **Self-Compassion Meditation:** Sit in a comfortable position and put your hands on your heart. Breathe a few times and say phrases like "May I be kind to myself," "May I be strong," and "May I find peace."

This exercise helps develop self-compassion, which is crucial in balancing your emotions during tough times. When you create a kind and gentle bond with yourself, you build a base of inner calm.

2. **Chakra Balancing:** This technique focuses on the body's energy centers, called chakras, to balance emotional and physical health. Sit and pay attention to each chakra, beginning at the spine's base and moving up to the head's crown. Picture each chakra as a spinning wheel of light, aligning and harmonizing as you breathe. This meditation can help to balance emotions, boost inner peace, and improve overall well-being.

3. **Sound Healing:** Make sound a part of how you ground and center yourself. Try singing bowls, tuning forks, or even humming. How these sounds vibrate can sync up with your body's energy spots. This helps loosen up tight spots, balance your feelings, and bring about a deep calm and relaxation. Sound healing works well to move stuck energy and let out emotions. The vibrations from these sounds impact your body's energy centers. This leads to tension, releases emotional balance, and creates a profound sense of peace. Sound healing is good at shifting energy that's not moving and encouraging emotional release.

Adding these grounding, centering, and visualization methods to your every day habits can greatly impact your stress management, emotional balance, and inner calm. Helping clients practice these exercises as a body-focused coach can give them the tools to build a stronger link with their bodies. This leads to more resilience and well-being in all parts of their lives.

Breathwork and Body Awareness Techniques

Breathwork and body awareness play a key role in somatic therapy. They provide effective relaxation methods, lower stress, and boost overall health. These practices help people link up with their bodies, let go of tension, and develop a stronger sense of being present.

Deep Breathing Exercises to Relax and Cut Down Stress

1. Diaphragmatic Breathing (Belly Breathing): Diaphragmatic breathing forms the base of somatic therapy. It helps people relax and feel less stressed by using the diaphragm, the main muscle we use to breathe.

- **How to Practice:** Get comfortable sitting or lying down. Put one hand on your chest and the other on your belly. Take a deep breath through your nose. Let your belly rise while your chest stays still. Breathe out through your mouth. Feel your belly go down. Pay attention to your belly moving up and down as you breathe. Do this for 5-10 minutes each day or when you're feeling stressed.

- **Benefits:** Diaphragmatic breathing turns on the parasympathetic nervous system. This system handles the body's "rest and digest" response. It can slow down your heart rate, lower your blood pressure, and reduce cortisol, the stress hormone. If you keep at it, you'll find it easier to manage your emotions and feel more relaxed overall.

<u>**Diaphragmatic Breathing**</u>

2. Box Breathing (4-4-4-4 breathing): Box breathing is a planned way to breathe that helps you focus, stay calm, and deal with stress better.

> **How to Practice:** Find a comfy spot to sit. Breathe in through your nose while counting to 4. Hold it for four counts. Let it out through your mouth, counting to 4. Pause again for four counts. Keep this pattern going for a few minutes, staying steady.

> **Benefits:** Box breathing helps control your body's automatic responses, reducing stress and worry. It's handy when you need to settle your mind and body fast, like before something stressful or when you're feeling anxious.

<u>**Box Breathing (4-4-4-4 breathing**</u>

3. Alternate Nostril Breathing (Nadi Shodhana): This old yoga breathing method brings balance to the left and right sides of the brain. It helps make your mind clearer and your emotions more stable.

> **How to Practice:** Sit up straight with a comfortable posture. Close your right nostril with your right thumb. Take a deep breath through your left nostril, then close it with your right ring finger. Open your right nostril and breathe out. Breathe in through your right nostril, close it, and then breathe out through

your left nostril. This finishes one cycle. Keep going for 5-10 minutes.

Benefits: This breathing technique balances the body's energy pathways and soothes the mind. It helps to lower stress, boost brain function, and support emotional stability.

<u>**Alternate Nostril Breathing**</u>

Guided Practices to Boost Body Awareness

1. Body Scan Meditation: Body scan meditation helps you become more mindful. It involves scanning your body with your mind to find areas of tension, pain, or relaxation.

> **How to Practice:** Lay down or sit in a comfortable position. Shut your eyes and take a few deep breaths. Start by putting your attention on your toes and move it up through your body—feet, legs, belly, chest, arms, and head. Be aware of any tight or uncomfortable spots without judging them. Breathe into these areas, allowing them to relax and let go. Keep scanning until you reach the top of your head.

> **Benefits:** Body scan meditation makes you more aware of how your body feels and helps you find areas where you might be holding tension or emotional stress. If you do this often, you can get more in touch with your body and get better at handling physical and emotional discomfort.

2. Progressive Muscle Relaxation (PMR): PMR influences reducing physical tension and heightening body awareness. This method involves tightening and loosening various muscle groups.

> **How to Practice:** Find a comfy spot to sit or lie down. Begin with your feet muscles. Tighten them, hold for a moment, and then let go. Work your way up to your calves, thighs, belly, arms, and face. Tighten and loosen each muscle group. Pay attention to how tension and relaxation feel different.

> **Benefits:** PMR helps to ease muscle tension, lessen worry, and boost body awareness. It works well for people who deal with ongoing tension or pain from stress.

Progressive Muscle Relaxation

3. Sensory Awareness Practice: This practice centers on the five senses to boost body awareness and root you in the present moment.

> **How to Practice:** Find a quiet spot and sit in a comfy position. Take a few deep breaths to center yourself. Start by looking at what's around you—spot the colors, shapes, and light in your surroundings. Then, listen to what you can hear, paying attention to sounds that are close by and far away. Next, feel the texture of your clothes or the surface you're sitting

on. Move on to smell and taste, even if these senses aren't as active. Spend some time on each sense, just noticing without making any judgments.

Benefits: Being aware of your senses helps you stay in the present, reduces worry, and makes you feel more connected to your body. This practice also makes you more mindful and can calm you down when things get stressful.

<u>Sensory Awareness Practice</u>

Combining Breathwork with Gentle Movement for Holistic Benefits

1. Yoga with Breath Awareness: Yoga mixes movement and breathwork to create a well-rounded practice. This practice boosts physical flexibility, clears the mind, and balances emotions.

How to Practice: Start with easy yoga poses such as Cat-Cow (Marjaryasana-Bitilasana) or Child's Pose (Balasana). While you do each pose, pay attention to your breathing—breathe in when you stretch or open your body, and breathe out when you contract or fold. Keep your breathing slow and steady, matching each movement to your breath.

Benefits: Yoga with breath awareness helps your mind and body work together, which lowers stress and helps you relax. Moving and breathing together boosts blood flow, eases tension, and calms your nerves. This leads to feeling better overall.

2. Tai Chi or Qigong: These old practices mix slow, careful movements with deep breathing. They help improve balance, flexibility, and relaxation.

> **How to Practice:** Start with simple Tai Chi or Qigong moves, like "Wave Hands Like Clouds" or "Gathering Qi." Match your breath to your actions—breathe in when you gather energy or move up, and breathe out when you release or move down. Make your moves smooth and ongoing, letting your breath guide you.

> **Benefits:** Tai Chi and Qigong boost physical balance, sharpen body awareness, and help you relax. Mixing breathwork with movement helps clear stuck energy, reduce stress, and create a feeling of balance and calm.

Tai Chi or Qigong

3. Walking Meditation: Walking meditation blends mindful breathing with walking, resulting in a moving meditation that anchors you in the present. This practice impacts your awareness, allowing you to focus on each step and breathe.

> **How to Practice:** Find a quiet spot where you can walk without interruption. Start walking at a slow pace, noticing how your feet feel as they touch the ground. Match your breathing to your steps—breathe

in for a few steps, then breathe out for the same number. Keep your mind on the beat of your movement and breath letting your thoughts clear as you walk.

Benefits: Walking meditation helps you stay in the present, reduces stress, and makes you feel more connected to your body. It's an easy but powerful way to bring mindfulness into your everyday life, boosting your physical and mental health.

Walking Meditation

Making breathwork and body awareness techniques part of your daily routine will create a stronger bond with your body, reduce stress, and boost your overall well-being. These methods help you deal with everyday stress and make you more resilient and able to handle life's ups and downs with more calm and focus. These practices impact your immediate stress levels and long-term ability to cope with challenges.

Chapter 6
Case Studies and Integrative Approaches
Real-life Success Stories with Somatic Therapy

Disclaimer: The names used in these case studies are aliases to protect the true identities of the individuals involved.

Somatic therapy has changed the lives of many people who face different challenges, such as sexual health issues, grief recovery, and chronic pain. The case studies below show how somatic therapy has helped people in real-life situations.

Case Study 1: Improved Sexual Health

Sarah's Story: Sarah, a 35-year-old woman, had trouble with low libido and intimacy issues in her marriage. She started somatic therapy and learned to connect with her body and emotions through mindful movement and breathwork. Sarah saw her sexual desire improve and her communication with her partner get better. She explored body awareness techniques and worked on underlying emotional blocks, which helped her sexual health and made her relationship stronger.

Key Techniques:

- Mindful movement exercises to reconnect with the body.

- Breathwork to handle anxiety and help relaxation.

- Somatic exercises to boost body awareness and intimacy.

Case Study 2: Grief Recovery

John's Journey: John, a 50-year-old man, felt deep sadness after his spouse died. Regular counseling helped a bit, but he still felt stuck. John tried body-focused therapy, which included grounding exercises, body-aware meditation, and easy yoga. These methods allowed him to process his grief more, leading to emotional release and a slow return to feeling normal.

Key Techniques:

- Grounding exercises to create stability and presence.

- Body-aware meditation to find and let go of stored emotions.

- Easy yoga routines to support emotional healing and help the body relax.

Case Study 3: Pain Relief

Emily's Experience: Emily, a 42-year-old woman, had chronic back pain that continued even after she tried many medical treatments. She started somatic therapy to understand how the mind and body connect and release physical tension through somatic movement and mindfulness practices. After a few months, Emily's pain levels dropped a lot, and she got back much of her physical function. She also learned ways to handle stress, which helped her manage her pain.

Key Techniques:

- Practices to become aware of the body to spot and release tension.

- Techniques to cut down stress based on mindfulness.

- Like the Feldenkrais Method, somatic movement therapies improve posture and ease pain.

Integrative Approaches for Comprehensive Healing

These case studies show that somatic therapy has a strong impact when combined with other treatment methods. For issues like sexual health, grief, or long-lasting pain, somatic therapy provides a complete way to heal by joining physical, emotional, and mental techniques. These people's progress highlights how important it is to tailor therapy and mix different approaches. This allows for a more profound and longer-lasting recovery.

Integrating Somatic Practices into Daily Life

Adding somatic practices to your everyday schedule can change your life, boosting ongoing self-care and maintaining somatic health. Here's how to make these practices a regular part of your life:

Tips to Add Somatic Practices to Daily Routines

1. **Kick-off Your Day with a Clear Mind:** Start your morning by taking a few minutes to breathe or do a quick body scan. This helps you stay grounded and prepares your mind and body for what's coming.

2. **Take Breaks to Move Around:** During the day, take short breaks to stretch, move, or do some easy yoga. Simple exercises like rolling your neck, shrugging your shoulders, or doing cat-cow stretches can help you release tension and keep stress from building up.

3. **Practice Evening Wind-Downs:** Before you sleep, do a relaxation routine that includes deep breathing or relaxing your muscles one by one. This helps you fall asleep more by calming your nerves and letting go of the day's stress.

4. **Mindful Walking:** Make your daily walk a mindfulness exercise. Pay attention to your breath and how your feet feel when they touch the ground. This easy practice keeps you in the present moment and works for any walk, whether you're in nature or the city.

5. **Turn Transitions into Chances to Practice:** Times when you're waiting or stuck, like standing in a queue or sitting in a traffic jam, can become moments to try

grounding or mindful breathing. This helps you stay balanced and reduces stress as you go about your day.

Making Custom Plans to Suit Each Person's Needs

1. **Figure Out What You Need and Wa nt:** Begin by pinpointing specific areas where you could use help, like handling stress, sleeping better, or easing body tension. Shape your body-centered practices to tackle these issues.

2. **Create a Plan That Fits Your Day:** Consider your daily schedule and spot times when you can add body-centered practices. This might be during your morning routine, lunch break, or before you hit the sack. The main thing is to make these practices regular and doable.

3. **Get Help from Tools:** Bring in tools like meditation apps, recorded guides, or yoga videos to give structure to your practice. Put reminders on your phone or calendar to nudge you to practice often.

4. **Flexibility is Key:** Being consistent matters, but give yourself room to change your routine when needed. Your life d oesn't stay the same, so your self-care shouldn't either. The aim is to make these practices a normal part of your day, not something you feel forced to do.

Why Taking Care of Yourself and Your Body Matters

1. **Self-Care as a Foundation:** Somatic practices you do often build the base for good self-care. They help you stay in tune with what your body needs and tells you. When you keep paying attention to your body, you can stop burnout, handle stress better, and feel good in the long run.

2. **Mind-Body Connection:** Keeping your body healthy ensures your mind and body stay linked. This lets you control your emotions better, bounce back easier, and stay healthier overall. This link matters a lot when you need to handle tough stuff in life.

3. **Preventative Health:** Using these methods often helps to stop stress and tension from building up. This build-up can cause physical problems and emotional issues. Making body-focused practices part of your daily routine makes you more resilient. You also keep a sense of balance and harmony.

4. **Long-Term Commitment:** Ongoing self-care isn't just about fixing current issues. It's a long-term promise to your health and well-being. When you prioritize body-focused practices, you invest in your future self. This ensures you stay healthy, balanced, and tough over time.

Making somatic practices a part of your everyday routine, setting up a custom plan, and sticking to ongoing self-care can build a balanced, tough, and healthy life. These methods aren't just for handling stress or unease—they're vital to living a grounded and satisfying life.

Making Your Own Somatic Therapy Plan

To make your own somatic therapy plan, you need to think about what you want, what you need, and how you live. Here's a guide to help you create a plan that fits you:

How to Figure Out What You Need and Want

1. **Spot Your Main Issues:** Start by pinpointing the key areas you want to work on, like stress, worry, lasting pain, or feeling more balanced.

    o   **Ask Yourself:** Which body feelings or symptoms bother you most? What emotions or thoughts come with these sensations? What kind of changes do you want?

2. **Make Clear Targets:** Decide what you hope to gain from somatic therapy.

    o   **Target Examples:** Lower muscle tightness, handle stress better, sleep better, bounce back from emotions easier, or know your body better.

3. **Look at Your Current Life:** Think about your daily routine, how much energy you have, and what you're already committed to.

●   **Factors to Think About:** How much time can you set aside for body-focused exercises? What parts of the day are you most likely to do these exercises?

4. **Pick Suitable Exercises:** Choose body-focused techniques that match your needs and goals.

   o **Some Ideas:** If you want to handle stress better, try breathing exercises and mindfulness. For ongoing pain, look into movement therapies like Feldenkrais or yoga that focus on body awareness.

Making Your Own Custom Plan

1. **Daily Practices:**

   o **Morning:** Begin with exercises to ground yourself or breathe to kick off your day on a good note.

   o **Midday:** Take short breaks to move or scan your body to ease tension.

   o **Evening:** Finish your day with ways to relax, like loosening your muscles bit by bit or doing some easy yoga moves.

2. **Weekly Practices:**

   o **Yoga Sessions:** Plan weekly 2-3 yoga or body movement sessions. Focus on spots that feel tight or help you let out emotions.

   o **Meditation:** Add 1-2 times where you scan your body or practice being mindful. This helps you understand your body better and handle your feelings.

3. **Monthly Review:**

●   **Check Your Progress:** Check how you feel in body and mind, and see if you're hitting your targets.

o   **Change Things Up:** Tweak your routine if needed. You might add new stuff or do things more or less often based on how you're doing and what you need now.

Checking and Tweaking the Plan Often

1. **Track Your Experience:** Keep a journal of your body-based practices. Note any shifts in how you feel. This helps you understand what works and what you might need to change.

2. **Set Periodic Check-Ins:** Plan regular times, maybe once a month, to think about your progress. Ask yourself:

o   **Questions to Consider:** Are my symptoms getting better? Do I feel more in tune with my body? Is there a specific practice that seems helpful or tough?

3. **Stay Flexible:** Be ready to tweak your plan as you grow. Your life, stress, and health needs change, so make sure your body therapy plan can change, too.

4. **Seek Guidance:** If you're unsure about any part of
    your plan or don't see the progress you want, think
    about talking to a somatic therapist to get advice
    tailored to you and make changes.

If you stick to these steps and keep up with your personal
body-based therapy plan, you can build a lasting and useful
way to improve your overall health. This method tackles
current issues and helps you stay healthy and strong in the
long run.

Conclusion

This guide has looked at how somatic therapy can help people. It covers everything from grounding exercises to personalized therapy plans. We've seen how it can make a difference to your body, emotions, and spirit. Somatic therapy brings together the mind and body. It gives you ways to handle stress, pain, and emotional problems. You can do this through mindful practices like breathing exercises, movement, and meditation. When you use these methods every day, you can become more resilient. You'll also understand yourself better. In the long run, you'll find more balance and healing. Make these practices part of your daily life. This way, you'll take care of your whole self.

⭐ Personalized Somatic Practice Plan – To-Do List ☑

Morning Routine:
1.Mindful breathing (5 minutes): Start your day with deep diaphragmatic breathing to set a calm tone.
2. Body Scan Meditation (5 minutes): Practice a quick body scan to identify and release any tension.

During the Day:. Movement Breaks (2-3 times/day): Take short breaks to stretch or do gentle yoga (e.g., Cat-Cow, Child's Pose).. Mindful Walking (10-15 minutes): Incorporate mindfulness into your walk, focusing on your breath and steps.

Evening Wind-Down:. Progressive Muscle Relaxation (10 minutes): Release the day's tension by tensing and relaxing muscle groups.. Evening Grounding (5 minutes): End your day with a grounding exercise, such as the 5-4-3-2-1 technique.

Weekly Practices:. Yoga Session (2-3 times/week): Practice a gentle yoga sequence focused on relaxation and body awareness.. Somatic Movement Exploration (1-2 times/week): Engage in freeform movement or dance to release emotions and connect with your body.

Ongoing Self-Care:. Journaling: Reflect on your somatic practices and any changes in your physical or emotional state.. Adjust as Needed: Review and adjust your routine based on your current needs and life circumstances. Flexibility is key.

Monthly Check-In:. Review Progress: Assess the effectiveness of your routine and make necessary adjustments.. Seek Support: Consider scheduling a session with a somatic therapist for deeper exploration or guidance.
This plan is designed to be flexible and adaptable, allowing you to incorporate somatic practices into your daily life in a sustainable way.

www.ingramcontent.com/pod-product-compliance
Lightning Source LLC
Chambersburg PA
CBHW050831250726

48653CB00006B/2549